for the one I love

- **04** PREFACE
- **06** WHY DADDIES NEED MUSCLES
- **07** HOW DADDIES GAIN MUSCLES
- **08** ALL YOU NEED FOR THE DADDYFIT TRAINING
- **10** A STRONG FATHER-CHILD RELATIONSHIP
- **12** SAFETY FIRST
- **14** DADDYFIT TRAINING
- **40** DADDYFIT WORKOUTS
- **44** NUTRITION
- **52** THE TEAM BEHIND DADDYFIT

CONGRATS, YOU'RE A DADDY NOW.

You are going to spend lots of time with your offspring. Time you used to spend doing all kinds of hullabaloo or sports.

Because their life is now changing, physical stress increases and time for sports runs short, many fathers tend to gain weight – 8 to 10 pounds on average during the first few years.

DaddyFit shows you how to use the valuable time you spend with your child for your workout too.

In cooperation with a personal trainer, a psychologist and a midwife, we developed a workout programme that is fun to do, works out your body and, at the same time, strengthens the relationship between you and your child.

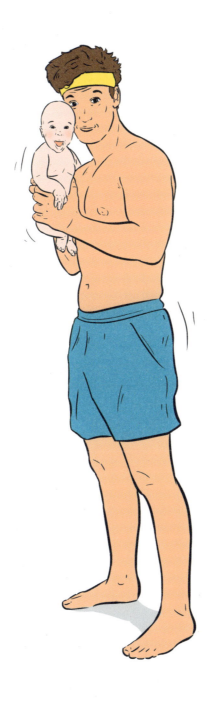

WHY DADDIES NEED MUSCLES

After birth, your baby is as light as a feather and you can easily carry it around for hours without losing that nonchalant facial expression of yours. But, day after day, it will become heavier, your biceps will start twitching, and that nonchalant expression will be replaced by a stressed one. Not cool. You will need power to keep your cool now.

But there are more reasons:

Strong muscles improve your metabolism, burn fat and create energy. They warm your body, support your brain function and improve your mental activity. Strong muscles strengthen your immune system and protect your internal organs. Sports and the associated muscle-building help to make you feel more balanced and happier. Maybe it will have the same effect on your wife, too ;)

HOW DADDIES GAIN MUSCLES

In order to achieve the maximum possible benefits from training and to avoid the risk of injury, a clean, focused and sensible execution is vital.

You should max out and – even if it hurts – exceed your limits with every exercise as long as your child allows you to. This will stimulate your muscles, make them angry and let them grow.

Furthermore, you should follow a balanced diet and give your body enough recovery time between exercises for your muscles to relax. Because, just like your child, they need sleep if you want them to grow.

ALL YOU NEED FOR THE DADDYFIT TRAINING:

A FITNESS DEVICE THAT GROWS ALONG WITH YOU AND MAKES YOU HAPPY.

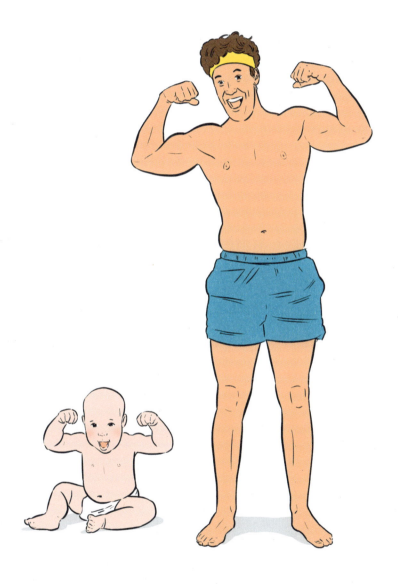

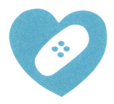

A STRONG FATHER–CHILD RELATIONSHIP IS A MATTER OF TRAINING

A bond is an invisible tie connecting two people to one another. An important part of shaping this attachment behaviour takes place within the first two years of a child's life. DaddyFit helps to playfully establish this invisible tie by making daddies spend lots of time with their offspring.

Science believes that babies and toddlers who can build on communion, closeness, security and the care of their parents right from the start develop a sense of basic trust for their future life, making them healthier, more caring, more stress-resistant, and happier.

But this valuable time spent together is not only good for the little ones. The physical and emotional closeness also strengthens daddy, because strong relationships between people are the basis for vitality and security. And that's a fact.

Tops off!
We recommend that both daddy and baby do the DaddyFit training topless. It looks good and feels even better. Skin on skin creates trust and a feeling of security. In addition, the vibration of the body and daddy's voice make sure that the baby feels safe and sound on daddy's chest.

You will find even more interesting facts on bonding with the respective exercises.

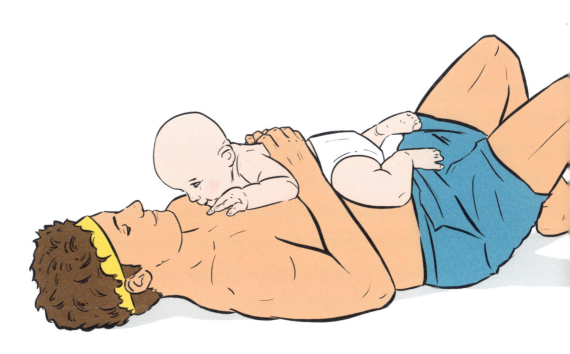

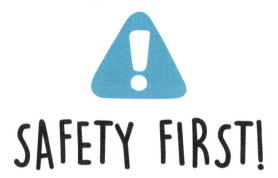

SAFETY FIRST!

Even though it is a known fact that daddies never need instructions, we simply have to make an exception to the rule here.

Some of the DaddyFit exercises should only be done when your baby is old enough and strong enough to support its body on its own.

In case anything is unclear or exercises somehow do not feel right, please skip the exercise and ask a doctor.

It's generally known that newborns and children don't like abrupt or quick actions. So please always be gentle, especially since your child has no control over its body at all.

From experience, we know that the little ones have lots of fun doing the DaddyFit training. In case you notice contrary signs from your child, please stop the exercise immediately and continue later.

DADDYFIT – SAFETY FIRST! 13

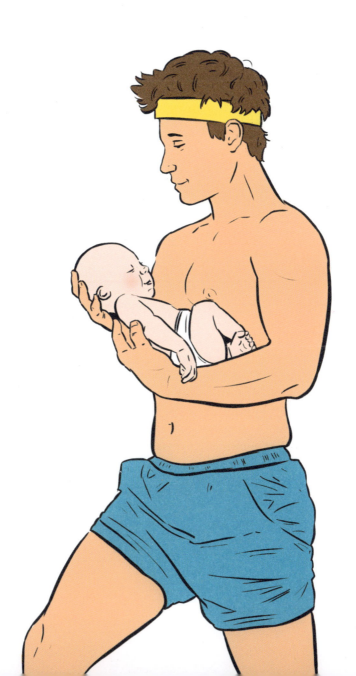

THE TRAINING

01 THE EXERCISE
SMOOCHY PUSH-UP
3 SETS AT 9–12 REPETITIONS

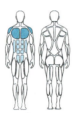

Smoochy Push-Ups – or push-ups, as childless people call them – especially strengthen your chest, shoulders, triceps and your baby's laughing muscles.

INSTRUCTIONS:
Lay your kid down on its back in front of you and lean over it with your hands a shoulder's width apart. Then lower yourself down until you can smooch your baby's belly. Push yourself up again and repeat until one of you can't take it anymore.

SAFETY FIRST

Even though the giggling will keep you going, make sure not to collapse onto your child.

Simply change from your feet to your knees when you feel the power disappear. After all, nobody will see it anyway and you can add some more smooches on top.

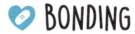 BONDING

Your baby will love this exercise. It will memorise your face and keep in mind who makes it laugh.

You will look forward to the next training and the time together will bond you together.

DADDYFIT – THE EXERCISE SMOOCHY PUSH-UP   17

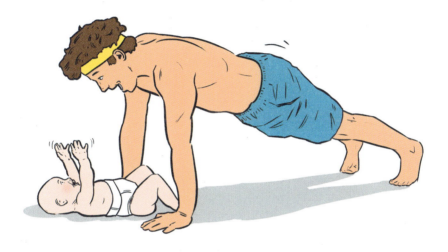

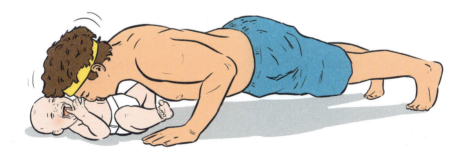

02 THE EXERCISE
WORLD CHAMPION
↻ 3 SETS AT 9–12 REPETITIONS

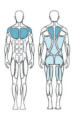 This workout exercises your bottom, your thighs and especially your shoulders, which looks good, of course.

INSTRUCTIONS:
Get into a stable position. Hold your baby face-to-face in front of your hips. Lift it up to eye level with your arms bent slightly and without swinging your body, kiss it on the forehead and lift it up into the night sky like you've just won the world cup. Lower your baby carefully again down to your hips and repeat the exercise until the next championship win or until you are too tired.

SAFETY FIRST

It is crucial that your child is able to look straight forward and hold its head on its own. That's why you should only do this exercise after the first six months.

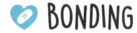 BONDING

Your baby feels that it can trust you, even high up above your head. You create a sense of basic trust which is essential for winning the world cup.

DADDYFIT – THE EXERCISE WORLD CHAMPION 19

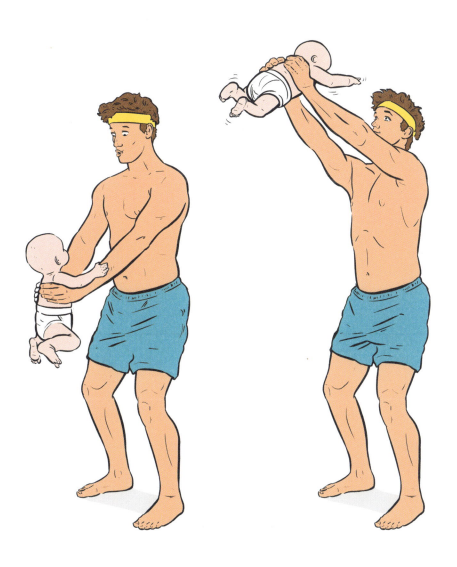

03 THE EXERCISE
AERO-PRESS
3 SETS AT 9–12 REPETITIONS

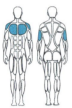

This exercise is for a wide chest, strong shoulders and defined triceps.

INSTRUCTIONS:

Lie down on your back with your baby on your chest and place your feet firmly on the floor. Slowly lift up your offspring into the air until your arms are fully stretched out. Hold it for a few seconds before preparing for a safe landing back on your chest. Repeat until one of you is too tired.

 ### SAFETY FIRST

Hold your baby tightly under the arms and make sure to carry out this exercise slowly.

Your child must be at least six months old, ensuring that it can support its neck on its own.

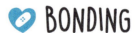 ### BONDING

Your kid will learn that there's very little in life to be afraid of and that you can always rely on each other.

DADDYFIT – THE EXERCISE AERO-PRESS

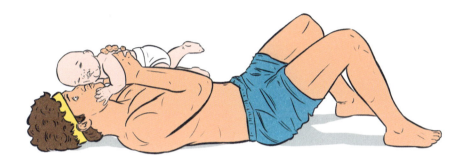

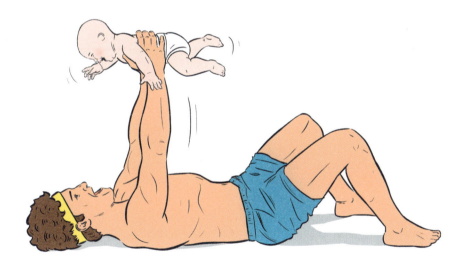

04 THE EXERCISE
BABY-CEPS
↻ 3 SETS AT 9–12 REPETITIONS

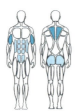

Baby-ceps will build good arms. You will need those, not only to look much better in a t-shirt – they will also help you carry your baby, who is getting heavier and heavier from month to month.

INSTRUCTIONS:
Stand with your legs a shoulder's width apart, your back straight and your knees bent slightly. Grab your baby under the arms making sure that you hold it safely. Lift and lower it slowly. Make sure not to fully stretch out your arms while lowering your baby.

 ### SAFETY FIRST

Like with all other DaddyFit exercises, it is important to securely hold your baby and carry out the exercise gently and slowly. Your baby will be ready for this exercise starting from six months of age. Only then it will be able to support its head on its own.

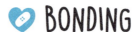

We have to be completely honest with you here: neither our psychologist nor the author have any idea on how this exercise affects the bonding.

Do you? Tell us on Facebook and, if it fits, we will include it in the next edition.

DADDYFIT – THE EXERCISE BABY-CEPS 23

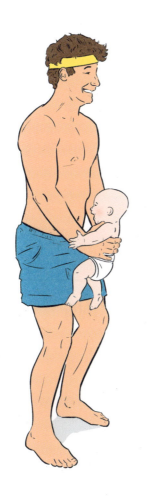
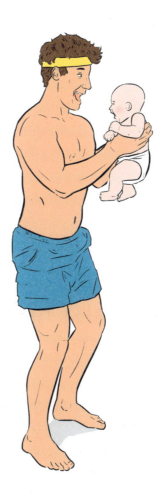

05 THE EXERCISE
PEEKABOO CRUNCH
3 SETS AT 9–12 REPETITIONS

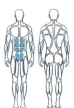

This training exercises your abs and once again the laughing muscles of your little one.

INSTRUCTIONS:
Lie down on your back with your baby on top of your chest. Legs bent and your feet in a stable position, a hip-width apart. Raise your head towards your chest and raise your legs. Hold this position before lowering your head and legs again. Repeat the "Peekaboo" until your abs shiver from exhaustion.

 SAFETY FIRST

Hold your kid tight so it won't scramble off your chest to cause an uncontrolled riot.

Your baby should be at least three months old in order to support its own body.

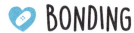 **BONDING**

This exercise is best carried out skin-on-skin with no shirts on.

It's the physical closeness, the skin-to-skin contact and the vibration of your chest that create a trustful feeling of security for your baby.

DADDYFIT – THE EXERCISE PEEKABOO CRUNCH

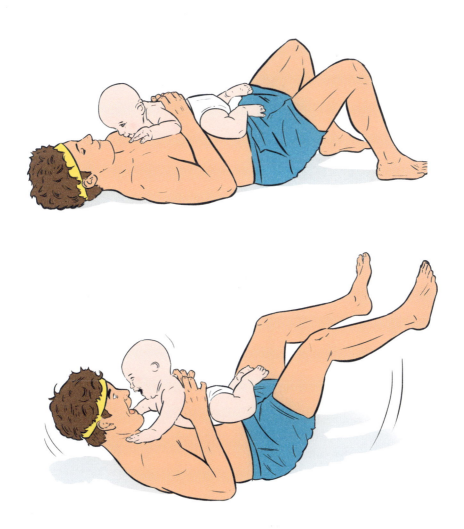

06 THE EXERCISE
DADDY PLANK
↻ 3 SETS UNTIL EXHAUSTION

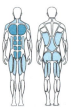

This exercise strengthens the musculature of your trunk, back and abs, as well as your baby's patience. Furthermore, you will find out who's the cooler one of you and winks later.

INSTRUCTIONS:
Prop yourself up on your elbows. Make sure that your feet are in a stable position, a hip-width apart and that your body is tense from head to toe, forming a straight line. Hold this position with a cool impression and keep breathing steadily. Even though it will sting, the sight of your loved one will ease the pain, like it always does.

⚠ SAFETY FIRST

Again, it is important to apply your strength correctly in order not to collapse right on top of your baby. Your kid will consciously notice you after the first six weeks.

🩹 BONDING

Your baby will learn how to be quiet with you and that life is not always about noise and hullabaloo.

Starting from the age of seven weeks, we are able to influence the development of our children's emotional spectre. It will exercise facial expressions and learn to interpret them, which could help to make out the fierce tigers in the urban jungle later in life.

DADDYFIT – THE EXERCISE DADDY PLANK 27

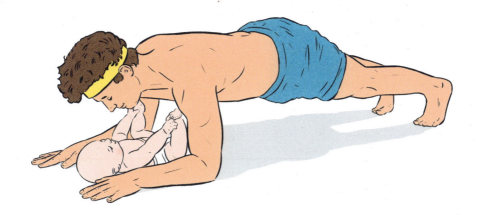

07 THE EXERCISE
SUPERDADDY
↻ 3 SETS AT 9–12 REPETITIONS

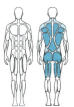

Superdaddy will give superpowers to your back, your bottom and your thighs, helping you to straighten out your body and relieve your spine.

INSTRUCTIONS:
Lie down flat on your belly. Stretch out your arms and legs to the front and back. Now hold your baby's hands and slowly lift them while lifting your own legs. The radius of movement is rather small, so try to hold the upper position even though it will sting and shiver. Superdaddy doesn't come for free.

SAFETY FIRST

Babies are able to sit from the age of eight to ten months. Until then, you will have to do the exercise while lying down.

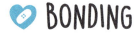 BONDING

Does your baby think it has superpowers because it can lift you up? If so, at least it won't damage its self-confidence.

DADDYFIT – THE EXERCISE SUPERDADDY

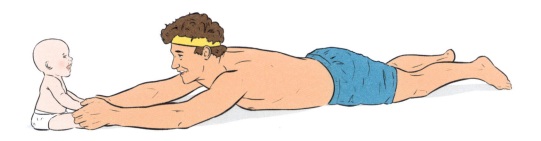

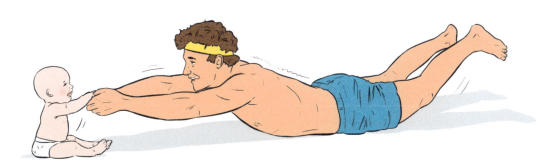

08 THE EXERCISE
BABY BRIDGE
↻ 3 SETS AT 9–12 REPETITIONS

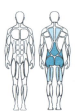

The Baby Bridge strengthens your whole back, allowing you to carry your child all the way through the park or the kitchen at night in style.

INSTRUCTIONS:
Lie down on your back with your feet a hip-width apart. Place your baby on your naked chest. Now tip your pelvis and start rolling up your back, vertebra by vertebra. At the highest point, your thighs and back will form a straight line. Only your neck rests. Roll back down again vertebra by vertebra.

⚠ SAFETY FIRST

Make sure to hold your baby tightly. Carry out the exercise gently and slowly, making it feel good and safe.

💗 BONDING

Baby skin on daddy skin is good for both of you. The bonding hormone oxytcin is released and strengthens your relationship.

The more you practise with your baby, the more solid your relationship will become.

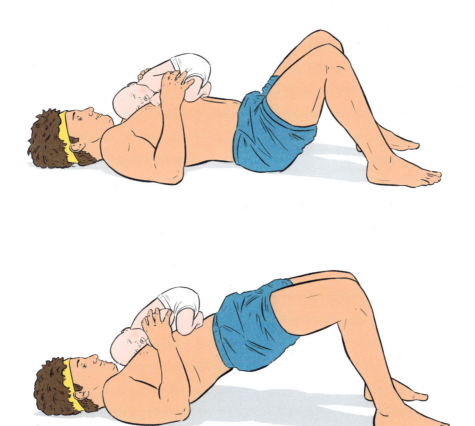

09 THE EXERCISE
DADDY SIT
↻ 3 SETS UNTIL EXHAUSTION

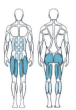

Daddy Sit strengthens your thighs, your bottom, your torso and above all, it looks really funny. This exercise can be easily done in the kitchen in the middle of the night and calms the both of you down.

INSTRUCTIONS:
Hold your baby in your arms and lean back against the wall. Now lower your body until your thighs and shanks form a right angle. Hold both your position and your baby for as long as you can.

 ### SAFETY FIRST

Be careful to hold your baby safely, especially when leaving the position.

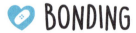

Same as with all DaddyFit exercises: tops off!

Since the bonding hormone oxytocin is also released when daddy's voice creates a feeling of security on a bare chest, counting or singing is another good idea – especially with your little one not yet able to distinguish between a 'good singer' and an 'okay singer' ;)

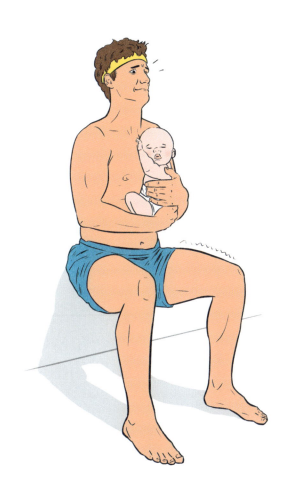

10 THE EXERCISE
DADDY SQUAT
↻ 3 SETS AT 9–12 REPETITIONS

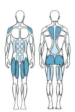

This exercise will especially benefit your bottom and your thighs. Mum's gonna be like 'Yum!'

INSTRUCTIONS:

Hold your baby tightly with your arms stretched out. Place your feet a hip-width apart with your toes slightly turned outwards. Stretching your abs and gluteal muscles stabilises your upper body and avoids a hollow back. Bend your knees until they are perpendicular to the floor. Push your body back up – slowly and in a controlled way – over your heels until your knees are almost stretched. Exhale while pushing yourself up.

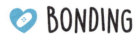

SAFETY FIRST

Make sure to hold your baby tight and safely.

Your child's neck won't be stable enough before the age of six months. Do not carry out this exercise at an earlier age.

BONDING

Your child will memorise your face. It can rely on it at any time and that strengthens the sense of basic trust to securely walk the path of life. Or better... fly!

DADDYFIT – THE EXERCISE DADDY SQUAT 35

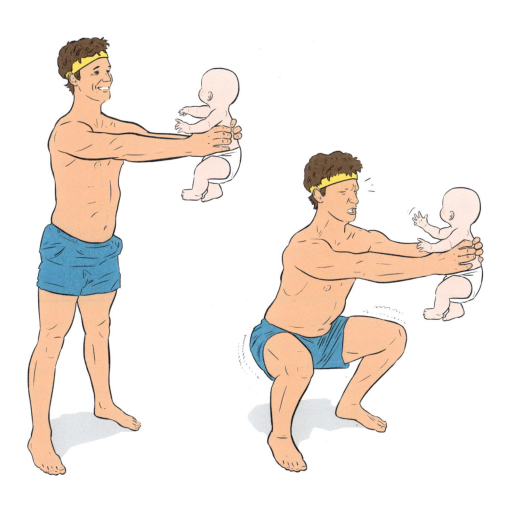

🔵 THE EXERCISE
STEP BY STEP, UH BABY
↻ 3 SETS AT 10 REPETITIONS PER LEG

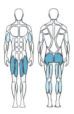 Taking big steps not only forms your thighs and bottom but also looks epic when strolling through the park.

INSTRUCTIONS:
Stand up straight with your feet close to each other, the tips of your toes pointing forward and your baby in your arms – heroic and secure. Gently place one foot forward, a bit more than a foot's length. Bend your legs until they reach an angle of 90°. Your upper body should be straight, with your back knee almost touching the floor. Get back into the starting position and repeat with the other leg – preferably until your baby falls asleep.

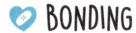 SAFETY FIRST
Make sure to hold your baby tightly and safely and to stand in a stable stance at all times.

💙 BONDING
Your baby is safely in your arms, feeling the warmth of your chest.

It enjoys the beautiful feeling of being carried in safe hands and that daddy is always there to do so.

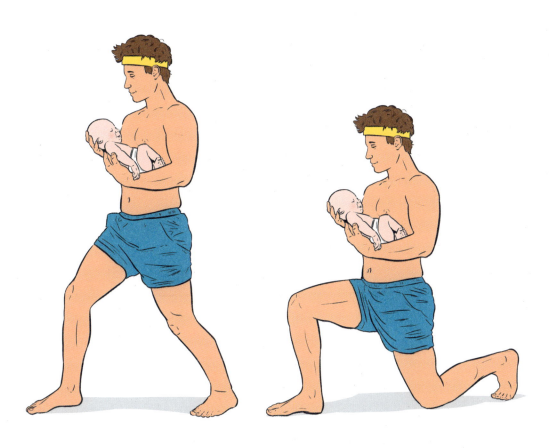

⑫ THE EXERCISE
THE EXPLORER
↻ OUT FOR A WALK 1–3 TIMES A WEEK

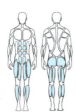

Running helps you keep a clear head – even in the rain.

Ask your kid. It hasn't learnt to moan about bad weather yet. Problems are solved while running. Daddies tend to be calmer. You train your endurance and your nerves. You will keep your cool for longer, even when a screeching scream abruptly ends your night's sleep.

INSTRUCTIONS:
Start with a relaxed run, walk for a bit and start running again. Once you notice it becoming easier, skip walking every once in a while. Simply forget about running. Think about other things. Once a week is a perfect start. Twice a week exercises your valuable endurance that comes in handy when carrying the pram up the dreaded stairs.

 ## SAFETY FIRST

Keep an eye on the traffic and make sure your kid sits dry and warm in the pram while seeing lots of the world around it.

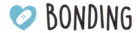

Daddy takes me all around the world while mummy has a little time for herself.

This also strengthens relationships ;)

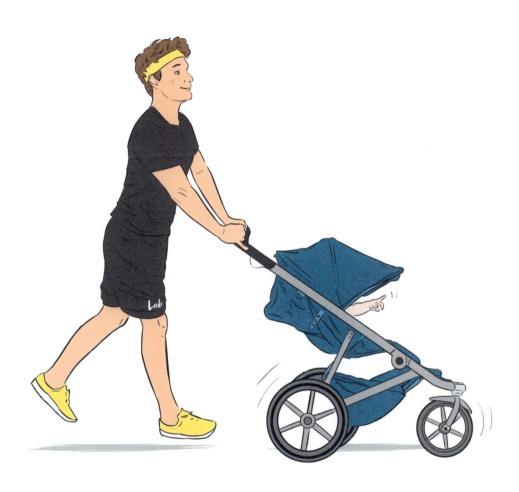

THE WORKOUT
LAZY BABY
↻ UP TO 4 ROUNDS

In case your kid is not in the mood for action, keep it busy with more passive exercises, while exercising your own body at the same time.

INSTRUCTIONS:

Carry out exercises 1, 2, 3 and 4 in a row as precisely as possible and repeat the set until you're tired. Please read the detailed instructions and descriptions before doing the respective workouts, even when you don't feel like doing them. It will pay off.

01 SMOOCHY PUSH-UP

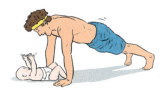
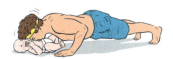

02 SUPERDADDY

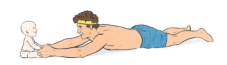
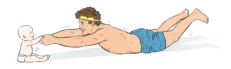

03 PEEKABOO CRUNCH

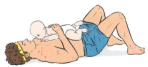
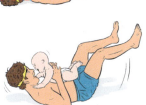

04 DADDY SIT

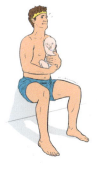

THE WORKOUT
ACTION BABY
↻ UP TO 4 ROUNDS

Let's say your kid fell into the druid's magic portion cauldron before birth or you notice that it needs that little bit of extra attention - try the DaddyFit Action Baby Workout, as it is the perfect way to play your kid to sleep. Maybe today both of you will sleep through the night :)

INSTRUCTIONS:
Carry out exercises 1, 2, 3 and 4 in a row as precisely as possible and repeat the set until you're tired. Remember: Please read the detailed instructions and descriptions before doing the respective workouts, even if men and daddies never really need instructions.

DADDYFIT – THE WORKOUT ACTION BABY

01 WORLD CHAMPION

02 DADDY SQUAT

03 BABY-CEPS

04 AERO-PRESS

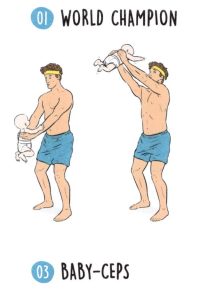
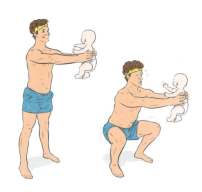
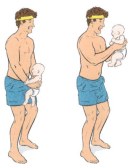
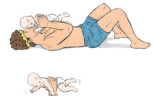
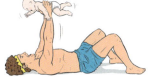

NUTRITION
DADDY'S FOOD

DaddyFit is not a book about nutrition. The topic is far too complex and every daddy eats completely different.

But daddies who strive for more power in everyday situations, and prefer to leave a soft baby belly to the babies, should follow some basic rules regarding nutrition.

No matter if you're a meat lover, vegetarian, vegan or even fruitarian: if you devour calories without burning them, you are bound to gain some sweet love handles yourself.

That's why this short chapter offers hungry daddies who never dealt with nutrition before some brief advice that might help you to be more aware of what you eat.

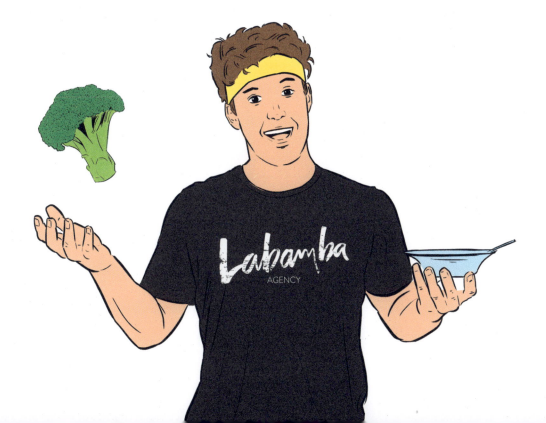

NUTRITION
LESS STRESS— MORE POWER

Everybody knows that a balanced diet can have a positive influence on body and soul. Good and healthy food calms us down and improves our well-being. It helps regenerate the body and build strong muscles that help us carry our babies a lot easier at the end of the day.

Daddies who partake in a mix of fresh vegetables, fruit, rice, nuts, fish, meat and dairy products (if necessary, vegetarian or vegan products depending on personal taste and belief), feed themselves with everything they need.

WHAT FOOD HAS TO OFFER

Apart from nutrients like vitamins, mineral nutrients, trace elements and important fibres, which, for example, make sure that this wondrous bowel of ours does what it does, we also consume further essential macronutrients.

Proteins. They saturate us, build up our muscles and allow them to grow when regularly exercised. If we would consume less protein than our body needs, it would feed on the protein from our existing muscles, causing them to shrink again.

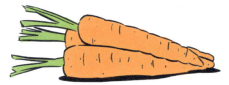

Carbs. They provide for our necessary energy and power that we need in everyday situations, to carry our little ones and fight through the third set of the DaddyFit Peekaboo Crunches.

Fats. They manage our blood pressure, have an anti-inflammatory effect, and are necessary for absorbing vitamins. Fats make sure we don't freeze and that our food tastes good. Besides, fats contain lots of energy. 0.002 lb of fat, for example, supplies twice as much energy as the same amount of protein or carbs.

LEAVING THE BABY BELLY TO THE BABIES

When daddies ingest more calories than they burn, their bodies store these calories as fat reserves. As long as daddies eat the amount of calories they burn, they won't gain weight. Sure, everybody knows that, but sometimes it helps reading it again ;)

A daddy weighing 176 lb, working in an office eight hours a day, burns approximately 2000-2500 calories. A daddy who is out and about all day working as a landscape gardener or a waiter burns around 3000–3500 calories.

On the following pages, you will find an overview of how many calories are hidden in various foods. All you have to do is add them up and you will gain a handy overview of your calorie stats each day.

Dig in!

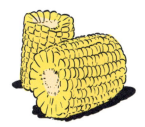

PROTEIN-PACKED FOODS, THAT FEED DADDY'S MUSCLES
CALORIES PER PORTION

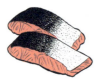

SALMON
One portion (0.45 lb)
= 376 calories

BEEF
One portion (0.45 lb)
= 214 calories

TURKEY BREAST
One portion (0.45 lb)
= 266 calories

CURD
One cup (0.45 lb)
= 216 calories

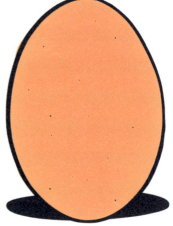

EGGS
One egg (medium, approx. 0.12 lb)
= 88 calories

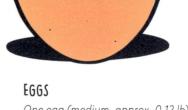

COTTAGE CHEESE
One cup (0.45 lb)
= 186 calories

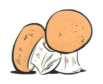

MUSHROOMS
One large button mushroom
= 4 calories

SOYBEANS
0,22 lb
= 446 calories

HIGH-CARB FOODS, THAT SUPPLY DADDY WITH ENERGY
CALORIES PER PORTION

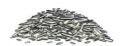

RICE
One portion (0.13 lb)
= 187 calories

PORRIDGE OATS
One portion (0.08 lb)
= 133 calories

CORN
One cob (approx. 0.33 lb)
= 129 calories

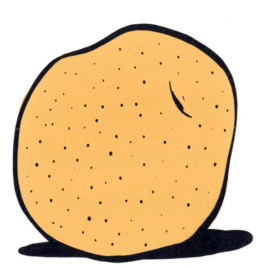

POTATOES
One large potato (approx. 0.2 lb)
= 66 calories

'GOOD' FATS, THAT SUPPLY DADDY WITH ENERGY AND HELP TO PROVIDE IMPORTANT VITAMINS

CALORIES PER PORTION

 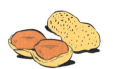 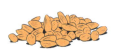

AVOCADO
Medium-sized avocado
= 365 calories

PEANUTS
One handful (approx. 0.05 lb)
= 145 calories

ALMONDS
One handful (approx. 0.05 lb)
= 153 calories

HIGH-FIBRE FOODS – GOOD FOR YOUR DIGESTION

CALORIES PER PORTION

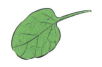 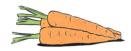 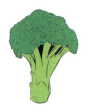

SPINACH
One portion (0.55 lb) =
68 calories

CARROTS
One carrot (approx. 0.17 lb)
= 25 calories

BROCCOLI
One broccoli floret
(approx. 0.77 lb)
= 119 calories

THE AMOUNT OF CALORIES IN DRINKS
CALORIES PER PORTION

MILK
One glass (0.2 l)
= 182 calories

COLA
One glass (0.2 l)
= 96 calories

CAPPUCCINO
One cup
= 50 calories

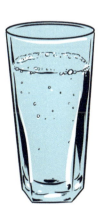

WATER
0 calories

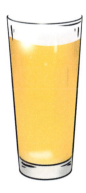

BEER
One glass (0.2 l)
= 95 calories

THE TEAM BEHIND DADDYFIT

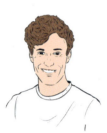

CHRISTIAN ROSENBROCK
PERSONAL TRAINER

For many years, Christian has been busy keeping his clients in shape. He contributed his knowledge to this book and impressed us all by modelling for our illustrator.

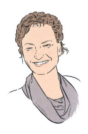

LISA BROCKMANN
MIDWIFE

Lisa knows how daddies should hold their babies because she has helped around 250 families to give birth to their children over the years. For years, she has also been counselling mummies and daddies after giving birth.

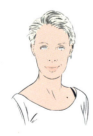

CLARA RÖDIG
PSYCHOLOGIST

Clara has been studying people's psyches and working with children and teenagers for over ten years now. Her expertise on father-child relationships has had a huge impact on this book.

DADDYFIT – THE TEAM BEHIND DADDYFIT   53

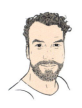

VAN DATA
STUDIO FOR ILLUSTRATION AND DESIGN

Michael, aka Van Data, dedicated his illustrational skills to the making of this book. www.vandata.de

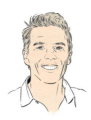

FELIX SCHULZ
AUTHOR

As of the date of this book's publication, Felix is neither a daddy yet nor lacking time and/or sleep – still, he gathered the combined knowledge of befriended daddies in DaddyFit.

The idea struck him when a friend told him that he didn't have time to do sports anymore and therefore slowly gained weight ever since becoming a dad. A year later, Felix handed him this book.

CONTACT

Have you ideas or tips on how to improve the training programme or the contents of this book?

What do you think of DaddyFit? Feel free to send us feedback and maybe we will include it in the next edition.
> **Facebook/DaddyFit**
> **hello@daddy-fit.com**
> **www.daddy-fit.com**

IMPRINT

All rights reserved.
No part of this publication may be reproduced, distributed, or transmitted in any form or by any means, including photocopying, recording, or other electronic or mechanical methods, without the prior written permission of the publisher, except in the case of brief quotations embodied in critical reviews and certain other non-commercial uses permitted by copyright law. All translation rights reserved.

Copyright © 2016 by Labamba Books, Felix Schulz Verlag,
Hamburg, Germany

First edition, 2016
Printing, binding and handling:
Schulz + Co GmbH,
Mühlenkamp 6c, 22303 Hamburg, Germany
Author, publisher, editorial, setting, design (including cover artwork), text, pictures, cover picture: Labamba Books, Felix Schulz

Illustration: Van Data – Studio for illustration and design
Cover design: Julia Günak / Wascooles
Graphic design: David Fischer
Printed and bound in Germany, 2016
ISBN 9783000535642

Please note:
The use of this book and the execution of the information contained within is at the user's own. The publisher and the author cannot assume liability for possible accidents or damage of any kind resulting from the execution of the excercises described herein for any legal reason. Liability claims against the publisher or the author for damage of material or ideally kind caused by usage or non-usage of the information and by the usage of incorrect or incomplete information are generally excluded. Claims and rights for compensation are therefore excluded. The work and all its contents were developed with great care. The publisher and the author do not assume any guarantee for currency, correctness, completeness or quality of the provided information. Print errors and misinformation can not be excluded. The publisher and the author do not take liability for printing errors or for currency, correctness or completeness of the contents of the book. The publisher and the author can not be held legally responsible in any way for incorrect information and consequences arising therefrom. All responsibilities for the contents of the websites mentioned in this book are exclusively on the part of the operators of the websites. The publisher and the author have no influence on the design or contents of third-party website. Therefore the publisher and the author dissociate themselves from all third-party contents. At the time of usage, no illegal content was present on the websites.